Plant-Based Eating
For Beginners

A Quick And Easy Solution to A Healthier Life

By **E.A. Rios**

For more information about

Weight Loss and Health visit…

https://www.30daybellyfatloss.com/

100% Free Report Reveals…

"How to Lose Belly Fat in 30 Days or Less With 25 Simple Tips"

Visit The Link Below To Get

Instant Access To Your FREE Report Now

https://www.30daybellyfatloss.com/

Disclaimer

This book has been written for information purposes only. In addition, every effort has been made to make this book as complete and accurate as possible.

However, there may be some mistakes in typography or content within this book.

In addition, this book provides information only up to the publishing date.

Therefore, this book should only be used as a guide.

The purpose of this book is to educate you about the Plant-Based Eating.

The author and the publisher do not warrant that the information contained in this book is fully complete and shall not be responsible for any errors or omissions.

The author and publisher shall have neither liability nor responsibility to any person or entity with respect to any loss or damage caused or alleged to be caused directly or indirectly by this book.

Table of Contents

Introduction

Many people panic at the idea of cancer, but the truth is that heart disease kills more people every year than the top ten cancers combined.

Every year, around 390,000 men and 271,000 women will have a heart attack. In addition, fifty-percent of women will die within a year of having a heart attack.

If you care about your own health, or that of someone you love, it's time to start living a healthier lifestyle.

And guess what?

A healthier lifestyle will be protective against many illnesses including cancer.

This wonderful eBook will guide you through the process of transforming your life and live a healthier lifestyle by eating a plant-based diet.

Although some people may think that a plant-based diet consists of eating nothing but plants, this is completely false.

Instead, plant-based eating can simply mean to eat more plant-based foods which consists of eating more than just vegetables.

In addition, there are different kinds of plant-based diets such as the **Flexitarian Diet, the Nordic Diet and the Ornish Diet** to name a few.

But the one plant-based diet you will be learning about is the amazing **Mediterranean Diet.**

For quite of few years now, the Mediterranean Diet has proven to be not just the best plant-based diet, but it has also proven to be the best overall diet to follow.

This remarkable eBook will show you why you deserve to eat well and how to succeed with getting started with plant-based eating.

In addition, you will learn how to develop the habit of eating more vegetables in order to get the powerful vitamins and nutrients that these foods have to offer.

You will also learn in depth about the Mediterranean Diet, the Mind-Body Connection of a healthy diet and more!

Chapter 1 – Plant-Based Eating

What is Plant-Based Eating?

Plant-based eating is simply eating foods that are primarily from plants. These foods include fruits, vegetables, nuts, seeds, oils, whole grains, legumes, and beans.

Plant-based eating does not mean that you are vegetarian or vegan. In addition, plant-based eating does not mean that you cannot eat meat, dairy or fish.

Instead, plant-based eating simply means that you prefer to eat more foods that come from plants.

Success with Plant Based Eating

The **Mediterranean Diet** is an excellent example of what plant-based eating is.

Although the Mediterranean Diet is considered to be the best diet for **Healthy Eating** and for **Plant-Based Eating**, the Mediterranean Diet is also considered to be a **'flexible'** **diet**.

What this means is that the Mediterranean Diet also allows consumption of fish, poultry, eggs, cheese, and yogurt a few times a week.

Overall, the Mediterranean diet offers amazing health benefits such as reducing the risk of heart disease, lowering diabetes and preventing certain cancers.

7 Ways To Eat More Plant-Based Foods

Here are some tips to help you get started on a plant-based diet:

1. **Eat more vegetables.** Simply include eating more vegetables in ALL of your meals and this includes breakfast.

    Also, eat a variety of colorful vegetables and make every effort to make your vegetables delicious.

    For example, you can make a **delicious vegetable smoothie** by using a combination of fruits and vegetables.

You can also use a **variety of salsas and spices** to add flavor to your vegetables.

2. **Reduce meat consumption.** Simply eat less meat and limit how often you eat meat in a month. Also, use **chicken, tofu and fish** as alternatives to eating meat.

3. **Eat healthy fats.** Healthy fats include Extra Virgin Olive Oil, salt-free nuts and seeds, and avocados.

4. **Cook primarily plant-based meals.** Build all of your meals around **beans, whole grains and vegetables.**

    You can even follow the **"80/20 Rule"** which means that 80 of your meals consist of plant-based foods and 20 percent of your meals can include foods that are not plant-based foods such as chicken, dairy or eggs.

5. **Include whole grains in your meals.** Start eating more healthy whole grain foods such as oatmeal, quinoa, brown rice and oats. Whole grain foods are full of fiber, reduce the risk of heart disease, fight off diabetes and prevent some forms of cancer

6. **Experiment.** Eat a variety of plant-based foods by trying and experimenting with new plant-based foods and meals.

   Eat a variety of plant-based foods by trying and experimenting with eating different vegetables, nuts, whole grains and seeds. Also, experiment by combing different plant-based foods at every meal.

   By experimenting with different kinds of plant-based foods you will come to realize that your meals become more delicious.

7. **Fruit and Nuts.** A quick snack or small meal can be a simple combination of fruit and nuts. Fruit and nuts are convenient and easy to eat especially when you are short on time.

How to Get Started with Plant-Based Eating

The Easiest way to get started with plant-based eating is to follow the Mediterranean Diet. The reason being is because the Mediterranean Diet is a very **easy and flexible diet** to follow.

In addition, research shows that the Mediterranean Diet is considered to be one of the healthiest diets in the world.

Another important point to mention is that although the Mediterranean Diet consists primarily of plant-based foods, it is a very healthy diet that anyone can follow whether you are a vegetarian or not.

For more information about
Weight Loss and Health visit…
https://www.30daybellyfatloss.com/

Chapter 2 - You Deserve to Eat Well

A lot of people seem to want to eat well, but tend to fall back into the same destructive habits.

While it may be confusing at times as to why this may be, the truth is that no matter how much we want to do things right for ourselves, it is difficult, if not impossible, if you do not fully believe you deserve to be taken care of.

Whether it is being taken care of by yourself or someone else, you do deserve to eat well. All of us have self-doubts at times, and some of them are so deeply rooted within us that it can lead us to act in destructive ways, whether we want to or not.

However, if we are willing to consider the fact that our self-perceptions are flawed, we can take the necessary steps toward healing those broken pieces of ourselves that make us stop believing we are worthy of being taken care of.

However, nothing that is injured within us is necessarily going to be broken forever. We can take the steps necessary to heal ourselves.

Even though that is difficult at times.

You have to be devoted to a path of self-healing before you can ever dedicate yourself to eating a nourishing diet if food is one of the things you use to punish yourself.

One thing that you can do to help yourself develop the self-love you need is to believe that you are worthy of a future full of eating healthy foods and free of disease and illnesses.

You can also practice other types of self-love, using methods such as mindfulness, journaling, meditation and using positive affirmations.

If you start a gratitude journal, you begin to take a close look at your life and see the things that you have to be grateful about.

When you are able to look at the positive things in your life, it can make it that much easier to see positive patterns and good things about yourself and the people you care about.

Not only that, but developing that **mind-body connection** is an essential part of learning to believe that you truly do deserve to eat healthy, nourishing foods.

You can also do meditation as a way to get centered within yourself and utilize mindfulness as a way of seeing the opportunities and beauty in every new day.

Mindfulness meditations help us to get closer to ourselves both inside and out and align with our true needs and desires, such as the need to be nourished, healthy and safe.

However, you choose to enhance your mind-body connection, whether it is journaling or meditation, they are all bound to help you to learn how to value yourself more deeply.

When you value yourself, you make decisions based on what truly fulfils you and as a result you will allow your body to thrive!

For more information about
Weight Loss and Health visit…
https://www.30daybellyfatloss.com/

Chapter 3 - <u>Why Some Diets Fail Us and What We Can Do About It</u>

Right now, there's a good chance that your daily diet is simply not good when it comes to ensuring you are in the best possible health.

In fact, there's a good chance that your diet may be killing you.

And what is the culprit here? The answer is **empty calories and processed foods.**

These days, a huge proportion of what we eat is already **prepared and 'processed.'**

That means that it has spent a lot of time in a factory and thus bears little resemblance to what the ingredients originally looked like.

A good example is a bag of chips, which doesn't tend to have much **real potato** left in it at all.

In addition, chocolate is made from a **cocoa beans** but the rest is purely processed.

And already made lasagna will have had all the healthy ingredients in it fried out of it and a ton of salt, sugar and bad fats added to it to try and keep it preserved.

All this means is that you're getting **'empty' calories** from your diet – calories that will provide you with energy and make you gain weight – but gain **no nutritional value** whatsoever.

Why We Need Nutrition

It is a mistake to think of food as fuel. Calories are fuel and they happen to be in our food, but food is more than just fuel.

Apart from also being a social event and a hobby, food should also be a source of **raw materials.**

The saying that you **'are what you eat'** is literally true and when you eat any meal, your body will break it down into certain parts and then reassemble those parts in order to build muscle, create enzymes and hormones and even produce neurotransmitters (the chemicals that make our brain work).

When you don't get these things, you'll find yourself feeling considerably worse.

For example, if you don't get enough **vitamin C** then your immune system won't be able to perform at its best and you'll be much more likely to get ill.

Worse yet, vitamin C is also crucial for helping you to produce **serotonin** (a chemical in the body that makes you Happy and helps you to sleep).

Take vitamin C away and your **mood and energy levels** will greatly decrease.

Similarly, when you don't get enough **omega-3 fatty acids** (healthy fats that help your body to function properly), it can cause inflammation in the body – this makes your joints hurt, creates "brain fog" and it can lead to illness.

In addition, a lack of **amino acids** (compounds found in foods that help the body maintain good health and function properly) will mean that your muscles are **weaker and smaller**.

And it will result in your skin looking grey and your nails being brittle.

Overall, your entire body will greatly be affected by having a lack of **amino acids** in the body.

These short-term **health problems/issues** can most definitely be something to worry about because they can negatively affect your health in the long term.

In addition, the damage from short-term health problems/issues are cumulative and in the end you will be more likely to suffer from a wide range of diseases and illnesses.

What to do About It

The answer is to stop thinking of food as fuel and to instead think about the **quality of the raw materials** you're putting into your body's system.

In addition, find ways to get more nutritious foods into your diet even if that means just adding a **smoothie** into your eating routine!

Healthy Eating – Your Future is *Now*

Sometimes, it seems impossible to make plans for the future, especially if you are insecure and find that when you do make plans, they never turn out quite how you expect them to.

This can create a sense of insecurity and anxiety in a person that can be difficult to overcome.

Whether you want to succeed or not, these seeds of doubt can plant themselves in your mind and prevent you from doing what it is that you want to do the most.

When it comes to your future, **healthy eating** is the most basic building block that will help you to **build yourself up** into something you have dreamed of being.

If you are not properly nourishing your body now, in the future, you are likely to suffer from it whether **emotionally, mentally or physically**.

Without getting the proper **vitamins and minerals** in the body (from eating healthy foods), you will ultimately find yourself suffering from debilitating diseases that could easily have been avoided if you were only more **conscientious** about the foods that you put into your body.

Believe it or not, but it can be surprisingly easy to live with **malnutrition**.

More specifically, you don't always realize that you are lacking in essential vitamins and minerals until you are suffering the consequences from it.

Sometimes, you can go to a doctor and they can administer to you (via prescription) the vitamins that you are deficient in so that you can begin to heal properly from it, but sometimes, that stops being an option.

Consider that **prevention** is the most important thing that you can do when it comes to sickness, illnesses and diseases.

Sometimes, you will never be able to cure what it is that you neglect such as your health.

And when the day comes that you are suffering for your mistake of neglecting your health, you will feel lost, confused and maybe even depressed.

Therefore, everybody needs to pay close attention to what they're putting in their bodies right now, because your future is **now**.

Something that can help you is looking into ways that your body needs to be nourished.

Look into your **body mass index** and see what it is that you should be eating every day nutritionally.

Start taking **multivitamins** daily just to make sure that you are never lacking in the most essential nutrients and minerals.

This is especially important if you are attempting to survive on a diet of processed foods and highly sugary beverages that make it almost impossible to lose weight.

If obesity is difficult enough for you to deal with, imagine finding yourself being diagnosed with cancer in the future because of processed food choices that you have made over healthier alternatives.

These are issues that can sometimes be avoided, and food can also act as **medicine** as much as prevention.

If you want to be healthy and happy, and you see yourself having a bright future, consider your **eating habits** as being very important for a healthy and happy life.

Therefore, makes **good food choices** in the present moment because your future is being built on every **choice and decision** you make today.

For more information about
Weight Loss and Health visit…
https://www.30daybellyfatloss.com/

Chapter 4 - <u>Develop the Habit of Cooking & Eating More Vegetables</u>

The standard American diet is generally referred to as a diet that is **lacking** in fruits and vegetables.

In addition, a lot of people don't go out of their way to eat fresh fruits and vegetables on a regular basis.

If anything, a lot of people settle for the kinds of foods that they can get in a **can**, and try to pretend that the French fries and their "Happy Meals" are nutritional enough as far as vegetables go.

Unfortunately, what you don't always realize is that foods such as potatoes are actually full of starch, which break down into sugar in your body and cause you to have rapid weight gain.

Potatoes are a **staple food** in many cultures, most notably the Irish, but the way that Americans prepare potatoes can make them very unhealthy to eat.

In addition, deep frying potatoes in oil is a sure way to obesity.

Instead of treating potatoes as your vegetable side dish for every meal, make sure that you have some **green vegetables** instead, or at least something that is fresh from the produce section on your table every day.

Consider that cooking fresh vegetables can be very tedious for somebody who is not used to the task.

In addition, you have to make sure that the vegetables are all washed and cut up and prepared before you even begin to cook them.

Therefore, it is no wonder why people who are used to the convenience of eating **processed foods** and the American lifestyle find themselves hard-pressed to make the time to prepare vegetables properly for themselves and their families.

However, there are some easier ways that you can **cook, prepare and eat** more vegetables on a daily basis.

If you want to transition into a healthy habit of cooking vegetables, there are some steps that you can easily take.

First of all, as soon as you buy your vegetables, **wash them and cut them up** so that they are ready for cooking once it comes time for your meal.

This will help to save you a tremendous amount of time in the long run, and when you take your vegetables out to cook them, you will be very glad to realize that you are making great choices for yourself and your family, if you are cooking for more than one person.

Next, it doesn't hurt to look into **recipe books and cooking videos** online.

If you learn how other people make vegetables and make them work in your favor, you can easily pick up **tips and strategies** that you need in order to make your vegetables taste good.

It is important to state that it can be very hard to break into a **new habit of cook, preparing and eating more vegetables** on a daily basis so be patient with yourself and don't try to rush it.

Finally, make eating more vegetables a **priority** in your life. Simply develop the habit of eating vegetables at every meal.

In addition, think about the vegetables that you enjoy eating and want to eat, and think about how you want to **prepare them**.

Consider that vegetables are **powerful natural foods** that are like medicine.

In addition, vegetables will protect you from **sickness, illnesses and diseases** and provide you with a clear path to a brighter, healthier future.

Getting Started with A Diet

When you have decided that you need a diet to supplement your body's nutritional requirements, you are deciding to make a **positive healthy change** in your life.

It is true that today we are not living as healthily as we used to.

Our foods have become more **synthetic** (created by chemicals).

In addition, the environment itself has become synthetic and our lifestyles have gone too far away from the order of nature to be considered healthy.

We are also too consumed with our **materialistic responsibilities** to realize our very own body's physical demands.

So, looking for a diet, a healthy diet and diet that is **sustainable** is a great idea.

But, if you have already started looking for diets, you might have understood that the whole process is not as easy as you think.

You are not going to find a single diet that is **perfect** in all respects that you can use for yourself without any short comings.

Simply, there is **NO Perfect Diet**. At the same time, you will see that there are hundreds of different diets out there and some are effective and others are not.

In addition, some diets can also be **expensive ones** and some diets are very **cost-effective**.

So, there are some diets that will treat you to **gourmet delicacies** even when you are dieting and there are other diets that believe in the old system of making the **body starve**.

In addition, one diet will tell you to keep away from one **particular nutrient or food group**, while another diet will tell you to keep away from another nutrient or a different type of food group.

Then you have the diet that has NO restrictions whatsoever.

Confused already?

If you are, it is not your fault at all. With the hundreds of diets out there, all of them with amazing promotional strategies and most of them with some great user reviews as well, it is understandable that you might find it difficult to find a diet that meets your **health and lifestyle requirements**.

In short, when you are looking for a diet, you need to check out the following things:

1. When a particular diet interests you, the first thing you should consider is the concept behind the diet.

    So, ask yourself the following questions regarding the diet:
    - "Why does this diet work?"
    - What principle is this diet based on?
    - What nutrients will this diet provide me with, and what are some food restrictions if any?

    These are the things that you have to look for in a diet.

    In addition, your choice of diet should always depend on the theory behind whether it is **healthy and sustainable**.

2. Your next step will be to get as much information as you can about the diet.

Visit some websites, read some books and ask some experts about the diet. Simply try to **learn as much about the diet** as you possible can.

3. Next, read some feedback about the diet. See how the diet is helping and affecting people who have used it already.

4. See if there are any drawbacks about the diet. Ask yourself, "Is there any reason why my body won't adjust well with this diet?

Now the one diet that has been proven over and over again to be effective at fighting of diseases and illnesses and has so many remarkable health benefits is the **Mediterranean diet**

Plain and simple, the Mediterranean diet is recognized by many experts to be the **Best diet for Healthy Eating, Easiest Diet to Follow, the Best Diet for Diabetes and the Best Plant-Based Diet**.

The Mediterranean diet helps with **weight loss, increases longevity and it is a very sustainable and 'flexible' diet** which means it can be used by anyone whether a person is a vegetarian or not.

For more information about
Weight Loss and Health visit…
https://www.30daybellyfatloss.com/

Chapter 5 - <u>The Mediterranean Diet</u>

The Mediterranean diet evolved over thousands of years and from different ethnic cultures near the Mediterranean Sea.

More specifically, The Mediterranean diet evolved as a result of the local people using their **immediate resources** to prepare food which resulted in The Mediterranean diet.

In addition, the food was based on the local culture of the people, the environment and the peoples personal beliefs and religious practices.

<u>The Mediterranean Diet for Beginners</u>

The Mediterranean diet is an **eating lifestyle** that follows the traditional way of eating in countries surrounding the **Mediterranean Sea**.

Such countries surrounding the Mediterranean Sea are **Spain, France, Italy and Greece.**

In order to practice the Mediterranean diet, it is important to learn about the exact foods that are consumed in order to benefit from the Mediterranean diet.

As stated before the Mediterranean diet is a lifestyle that consists of eating **whole natural foods such as fruits, vegetables, whole grains, legumes and olive oil.**

In addition, foods such as **red meat, pork and processed foods** are NEVER consumed in the Mediterranean diet. However, chicken and eggs are consumed occasionally.

Important and excellent protein sources such as **fish, seafood and lentils** (also contain a lot of fiber) are also consumed in the Mediterranean diet.

The Mediterranean diet also includes **high fiber foods** such as fruits, vegetables and legumes such as kidney beans and chickpeas.

Health Benefits of the Mediterranean Diet

Below are some important health benefits of the Mediterranean diet:

1. **Prevent strokes and heart disease.** This means eliminating **processed breads or foods** from your diet.

In addition, greatly reduce the amount of **red meat** that you eat. Also consider **eliminating alcohol** from your diet but moderate amounts of red wine are allowed.

2. The foods in the Mediterranean diet contain of a lot of **vitamins and nutrients** which are good for your **body, your brain, your heart and your bones**.

   As a result, the Mediterranean diet will help to reduce your risk of **Parkinson's Disease**.

   In addition, you will have more energy, feel stronger and younger, live longer and feel overall great.

3. Keeps your **brain sharp, alert and active** and helps prevent brain disease such as **Alzheimer's Disease and Dementia**.

4. Improves your **cholesterol and blood sugar levels**. In addition, protects you from diabetes and helps you maintain a healthy weight.

5. Improves your **memory and your ability to focus and concentrate**.

6. Improves **longevity** as a result of consisting of plant-based whole natural foods that provide powerful **antioxidants, vitamins and nutrients** essential for the body and mind.

7. Gives your body a lot of vitamins and nutrients which helps to **improve your mood and fight off depression as well as reduce stress and anxiety**.

8. Helps to fight off various kinds of **cancer**.

As you can see, there are so many amazing benefits of the Mediterranean diet as a result of the Mediterranean diet consisting of **whole natural foods** that provide the body and mind with powerful antioxidants, vitamins and minerals.

Food List for the Mediterranean Diet

1) **Eat Vegetables such as:**

Cucumbers, Broccoli, Carrots, Spinach, Kale, Celery, Cabbage, Collard Greens, Etc.,

2) <u>**Dairy (Drink and Eat Low Amounts and in Moderation) such as:**</u>

Greek Yogurt, Goat Cheese, ricotta cheese, etc.,

3) <u>**Rarely Eat Meat**</u>

If you do decide to eat meat try to eat Grass-fed beef.

4) <u>**Eat in Moderation Poultry and Eggs**</u>

If you do decide to eat poultry and eggs try to eat Organic chicken and eggs.

5) <u>**Definitely Eat Healthy Fats and Nuts such as:**</u>

Avocados, Extra Virgin Olive Oil, Walnuts and Almonds (unsalted), Flax Seeds, etc,

6) <u>**Eat Legumes such as:**</u>

Kidney Beans, Lentils, Chickpeas, Lima Beans, Black beans, etc.,

7) <u>**Eat Fruits such as:**</u>

Grapefruit, blueberries, Pomegranate, apples, etc.,

8) <u>**Eat Fish and Seafood such as:**</u>

Salmon, Sardines, shrimp, tuna, herring, shellfish, etc.,

9) <u>**Definitely Eat Whole Grains such as:**</u>

Brown Rice, Steel Cut Oats, Millet, Quinoa, Barley, Buckwheat, etc.,

10) <u>**Use Herbs and Spices such as:**</u>

Ginger, pepper, Garlic, oregano, parsley, basil, etc.,

<u>Mediterranean Diet Foods to Avoid</u>

- Refined grains, white bread, white flour.
- Refined oils such as soybean oil and canola oil.
- Foods with sugar such as sodas, candies, cakes.
- Deli meats, processed meats, hot dogs.
- Alcohol - red wine is allowed in moderation.
- Basically, any foods that are processed should be eliminated form the Mediterranean Diet.

* Remember, only **whole natural foods** should be eaten with the Mediterranean Diet.

Mediterranean Diet

Easy to Make - 7 Day Meal Plans

Day 1

Breakfast

Greek Yogurt with almonds and blueberries or strawberries

Lunch

Sardines with vegetables such as spinach or broccoli

Add some beans (black beans, kidney beans) for additional nutrients

Dinner

Chicken or Tofu with Quinoa and green veggies

Day 2

Breakfast

Whole grain oats with fruit (banana, berries) and mixed nuts (unsalted walnuts, almonds, cashews)

Lunch

Tuna with lentils and vegetables such as carrots and peas

Add additional green veggies for additional nutrients

Dinner

Salmon with mixed vegetables and Brown Rice

Day 3

Breakfast

Smoothie using Whole grain oats and veggies such as spinach. Eat with a handful of mixed nuts (walnuts, almonds or cashews).

Lunch

Tofu with lentils and vegetables and whole grain pita bread.

Dinner

Chicken breast with whole grain wraps and mixed vegetables (Chicken Tacos)

Day 4

Breakfast

Fruit with mixed nuts and whole grain millet.

Lunch

Avocado tacos using whole grain wraps, black beans, spinach, tomatoes and chopped bell peppers

Dinner

Mackerel (fish) cooked with olive oil, garlic, ginger. Eat with whole grain pasta and mixed vegetables

Day 5

Breakfast

Vegetable Omelet or scrambled eggs with vegetables (spinach). Include tomatoes and eat with whole grain Rye Bread.

Lunch

Spinach chicken salad. Add a variety of legumes like beans and chopped avocado for addition flavor.

Dinner

Sardines with whole grain bread dipped in Extra Virgin Olive Oil. Eat with mixed vegetables

Day 6

Breakfast

Whole grain oats with scrambled eggs. Include a vegetable spinach smoothie with blueberries.

Lunch

Tuna tacos using whole grain wraps. Add black beans and chopped avocado for addition flavor. Flavor your tacos with Extra Virgin Olive Oil if needed.

Dinner

Quinoa with shrimp. Eat with mixed vegetables

Day 7

Breakfast

Greek yogurt Smoothie with fruit and spinach.

Lunch

Scrambled eggs mixed with mixed vegetables and an avocado. Eat with whole grain bread.

Dinner

Chicken breast with lentils, beans and vegetables (broccoli and carrots). Use whole grain wraps if needed.

Mediterranean Diet Snacks and Desserts

- Unsalted Nuts or mixed Nuts (walnuts, almonds, cashews)
- Dried Fruits
- Greek yogurt
- Fruit (blueberries, apples, oranges, etc.,)
- Baby carrots
- Smoothie – (use whole gran oats, spinach and Greek yogurt)

Mediterranean Diet Food Pyramid

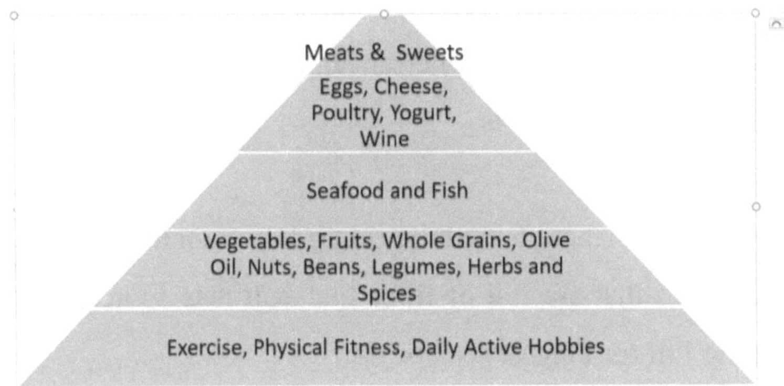

<u>The Mediterranean Diet and Weight Loss</u>

You will easily lose weight on the Mediterranean Diet because you will be eating whole, natural foods.

In addition, the Mediterranean diet consists of **healthy protein sources** and lots of **high fiber foods** which help to keep you feeling full.

The Mediterranean diet is predominately a **plant-based diet** that helps with weight loss, increases your lifespan and greatly improves your overall health.

In addition, foods such as <u>**sugar and processed foods**</u> are eliminated from this diet which tremendously helps to eliminate weight gain.

Plain and simple, the Mediterranean diet requires you to eat healthy nutritious foods.

Also consider that you will be eating **low calorie foods** like vegetables that are full of **fiber** that will help to keep you feeling full for long periods of time.

<u>The Mediterranean Diet Lifestyle</u>

The Mediterranean diet requires you to be "active" and to get some exercise and move around more often.

Actually, because you will be eating lots of whole natural foods, you will be getting a lot of vitamins that will give you lots of **energy**.

Therefore, you will feel more **energetic** and are going to want to naturally want to move around more often throughout the day.

Keep in mind that the Mediterranean diet is a <u>**lifestyle**</u> that requires you to eat whole natural healthy foods and eliminate processed foods as well as sugary foods.

In order to SUCCEED with the Mediterranean diet, you need to experiment with eating all kinds of whole natural healthy foods.

In addition, you need to experiment with **mixing** the types of foods that you eat with the Mediterranean diet so that you can make your meals delicious and rewarding to eat.

Therefore, don't be afraid to combine various fruits, vegetables, whole grain foods as well as spices and herbs in all of your meals.

Keep in mind that what makes any food delicious is **experimenting** with different combinations of foods, spices, and herbs so don't be afraid to experiment with the Mediterranean diet.

Also remember that the Mediterranean diet is not a "rigid" diet but more of a **lifestyle** that consists of eating whole natural foods and getting some exercise every day.

Mediterranean Diet

Foods to Eat Every Day

Vegetables, whole grains, fruits, legumes, nuts, seeds, extra virgin olive oil.

Foods to Eat in Moderation

Chicken, eggs, yogurt and cheese

Foods to Occasionally (Rarely Eat)

Red meat including beef, pork, sausages, etc.,

Foods to Never Eat

Processed foods, cooking oils and sugary drinks

How to Get Started FAST with the Mediterranean Diet

1) Add more green leafy vegetables to **ALL** of your meals. Simply eat them at every meal.

2) Eat good healthy fish a few times a week such salmon, tuna and sardines.

3) Eat healthy fats such as unsalted nuts (walnuts, almonds, etc.,), Extra Virgin Olive Oil and avocados.

4) Eat whole grain foods such as Quinoa, brown rice, oats, buckwheat, etc.,

5) Eat a variety of fruit every day. Consider making fruit your **dessert** at every meal. In addition, fruits can be used as good **snacks**.

To get started with the Mediterranean diet is quite easy. First, you want to keep your meal plans easy.

So, consider what fruits you like to eat and then make those fruits part of your meals or snacks.

So, if you like apples, blueberries and oranges then makes these your **"go to"** fruits which means you eat these foods whenever you are hungry.

Next, consider your **protein sources**. Good protein sources for the Mediterranean diet are salmon, tuna, sardines, legumes such as lentils, chickpeas and even chicken or eggs (eat occasionally) are a good source of protein.

Also consider using **tofu** as a source of healthy protein even though it is not part of the Mediterranean diet.

The Mediterranean Diet and Fitness

The Mediterranean diet is great for **fitness enthusiasts and athletes** because the whole natural foods that are consumed on this diet provide a lot of vitamins, nutrients and energy which are needed for **optimal performance** when doing exercise and in achieving certain levels of **physical fitness**.

In addition, the Mediterranean diet can **increase the athletic performance** of an athlete, specifically **endurance and strength**, because the Mediterranean diet is very rich in vitamins and nutrients which helps with nourishing the body with the necessary vitamins and minerals it needs for performing at **optimal levels**.

Also consider that the Mediterranean diet includes all the **healthy proteins, vegetables, fruits, healthy fats and carbs** that are necessary for any athlete to perform at optimal levels.

<u>The Mediterranean Diet vs Other Diets</u>

The Mediterranean diet has been considered by many doctors, researchers and experts to be a very healthy diet compared to other diets because of the simple fact that it only restricts **processed foods as well as sugary foods and drinks.**

Unlike other diets which restrict **healthy carbs like fruits and vegetables** or even healthy protein sources like **fish, chicken and eggs**, the Mediterranean diet **does not restrict** a person's consumptions of these foods simply because they have **nutritional value**.

What also makes the Mediterranean diet so great is that it is more of an **"eating lifestyle"** than a very strict diet.

So, there is no need to count calories or worry about feeling malnourished on the Mediterranean diet because you will be receiving a good amount of healthy proteins, carbs, fats and plenty of vegetables and fruits from this diet.

In addition, the Mediterranean diet can also be used with other diets which makes it a very **flexible diet** as well as a diet that any person can **adapt to and sustain** over long periods of time.

What also makes the Mediterranean diet so great is that there are so many combinations of foods, flavors and recipes that can be used for eating healthy, delicious meals.

In addition, the Mediterranean diet will help **with weight loss, improve your athletic performance and your overall health** and it is a very easy diet to sustain when compared to other diets.

The Mediterranean Diet Cost Effective

Eating healthy on the Mediterranean diet means you spend a lot **less money** on food.

More specifically, your grocery bills at the supermarkets come down drastically and you don't go into debt by going out to eat at restaurants as often as before.

In addition, you **save a lot of money** by not having to go to the doctor as often and having to pay expensive medical bills as a result of living a **healthy lifestyle**.

Mediterranean Diet Fights Toxins

A lot of foods nowadays are **toxic** because of the **synthetic chemicals** present in them.

When you're attempting to **eat healthier** by following the Mediterranean diet, you are less likely to get these toxins into your body.

What is great about the Mediterranean diet is that it requires you to eat **whole natural foods**.

So, the more whole natural foods you eat the **less likely** you are to get toxins to enter your body.

In addition, the Mediterranean diet consists of many nutritious foods that contain **powerful antioxidants** that help to fight off toxins from entering your body.

<u>Mediterranean Diet Provides Energy</u>

Because the Mediterranean diet requires you to eat whole natural foods, you will be getting a lot of **vitamins and nutrients** in your body.

This means that you will have a **lot more energy** to do more and achieve more in your life.

This **abundance of energy** will allow you to exercise more, travel more, play more, work more and therefore make your life more **productive**.

In addition, you will be able to **spend more quality time** with your family, friends and loved ones and that will surely enrich your life.

The Mediterranean Diet and Juicing

Overly cooking and processing of healthy foods **destroys** important micronutrients in healthy foods by changing their shape and chemical makeup.

The Mediterranean diet advocates that we eat a good amount of **fruits and vegetables** every day.

Now one way to make sure you consume a good amount of fruits and vegetables every day is by **juicing**.

Juicing is a simple way to easily guarantee that you **consume** enough fruits and veggies on a daily basis.

While you may surely juice fruits, if you're **overweight, have high blood pressure, diabetes or high cholesterol** it's best to limit juicing fruits until you normalize these health conditions.

The exclusion would be **lemons and limes** which have virtually none of the sugar, fructose that causes most of the metabolic ramifications.

Additionally, lemons or limes are great at **eliminating the bitter taste** of the dark leafy green veggies that supply most of the benefits of juicing.

<u>The Juice</u>

There are **2 main reasons** why you'll want to think about incorporating **veggie juicing** into your Mediterranean diet plan:

1) Juicing helps you to easily **drink** and **absorb** all the **nutrients** from veggies.

   This is important because you can quickly and very easily consume a large number of important **vitamins, nutrients and antioxidants** from vegetables.

2) Juicing helps you to consume a **wide variety** of **veggies** in a quick and easy manner.

   So instead of preparing, cooking and try to eat a large amount of vegetables every day, you can easily **juice** all your vegetables and **drink them** with all of your meals.

Simply by juicing your vegetables, you will be able to consume a wider **variety of veggies** into your diet.

It is important to eat a wide variety of vegetables because every vegetable provides different **vitamins, nutrients and antioxidants** to the body.

Now if you're new to juicing, there are many **economical juicers** to choose from.

Also, consider that juicing is not a chore but instead a more **pleasant** way of consuming more vegetables into your diet.

In addition, juicing vegetables is a lot **easier** than preparing and cooking vegetables to eat.

It is important to note that vegetable juice has **very little protein** and nearly **no healthy fat** so by itself it is not truly a complete food.

Therefore, vegetable juice should be used in **addition** to your regular **Mediterranean diet meals** not in place of them.

So, unless you're undergoing some special **fasting or detoxification** regimen it's likely unwise to utilize juicing as a meal replacement. Ideally **vegetable juice** may be ingested with your meals or as a between **meal snack**.

Below are a few easy examples of **juicing vegetables** to get you up and juicing fast:

First, make sure to use **pesticide free** vegetables. In addition, try to use **organic vegetables** if possible.

Here is a short list of some good vegetables to use for juicing:

- Celery
- Spinach
- Kale
- Collard Greens
- Red/Green/Romaine Lettuce
- Carrots
- Cucumber
- Endives

To give your vegetable juice some flavor you can use **lemons or limes**.

Lemons or limes are great for reducing the bitterness of certain vegetables such as Kale and Collard Greens.

In addition, you can even use a fruit like an **apple or a banana** with your vegetable juice.

Just make sure not to add too many fruits to your veggie juice because they contain sugar which can lead to some health problems.

The Rewards of the Mediterranean Diet

There are several benefits of following the Mediterranean diet. Below is a short list:

1) **Maintain a healthy body weight.**
2) **Maintain normal blood sugar levels.**
3) **Reduce the risk of heart attacks.**
4) **Reduce the risk of cancer.**
5) **Improves good blood circulation and maintains stable energy levels throughout the day.**

What makes the Mediterranean diet so great is that it requires you to eat a good amount of healthy **protein, fats, and carbohydrates**, which consist of lots of important vitamins, nutrients and minerals that the body needs.

As a result of following the Mediterranean diet, you will achieve the following **optimum health benefits:**

- More energy
- Improve mood and feel happier
- A boost in brain power - your memory will improve and you will be able to learn and process information better and faster.
- Reduction in stress
- Better focus and concentration

Simply by following the Mediterranean diet, you will be improving your **overall health**.

Remember, your entire body is **interconnected** so if you eat healthy foods this will affect your body, your heart, your brain and your mood.

Aside from improved health, you will develop **healthy habits and a healthy lifestyle** which can possibly have a positive influence on your family members and friends.

Also, keep in mind that as you follow the Mediterranean diet and begin to **lose weight, look younger and feel great,** there will be NO reason whatsoever to ever go back to eating unhealthy foods.

Succeeding with the Mediterranean Diet

Getting There: Targets and Objectives

You know that taking care of your health is important.

Creating the **right mindset** is the initial step to embarking on a **change** for the better that will allow you to prepare for the emotional struggle that is often associated with a **lifestyle adjustment**.

To complement all that **mental preparation**, you will secure your success by setting **milestones of achievement** that will be a motivational tool to help you reach your ultimate goal of a **healthy and active life**.

So, to achieve great results with the Mediterranean diet, it is important to **create a plan**, follow it through and keep track of your progress along the way.

A very common system for **setting and achieving goals** uses the acronym **SMART** as outlined below:

<u>SMART</u> stands for:
- Specific
- Measurable
- Attainable
- Rewarding
- Time-bound

****The SMART** acronym is discussed in more detail below:

1) <u>S</u>MART – 'S' stands for <u>Specific</u>

Be <u>specific</u> and define your **health/weight loss/nutrition/fitness goals** in a short direct statement.

For example, a <u>specific</u> weight loss goal is: **"My goal is to lose 10 pounds."**

2) SMART – 'M' stands for <u>Measurable</u>

Be sure your <u>goal</u> is something that you can <u>determine and measure</u>.

For example, write down, **"I will lose 10 pounds by October 1st, 2020"** as opposed to "I will lose weight."

3) SMART – 'A' stands for <u>Attainable</u>

You want to make sure you have a goal that is **"realistic"** and is <u>attainable</u> in order to build your confidence levels and to help you continue pushing towards your bigger goals.

For example, if your <u>major goal</u> is to lose **30 pounds**, then first begin with a <u>smaller</u> goal like losing **10 pounds**.

By starting with a smaller goal, you can set a **"realistic"** date for losing those first 10 pounds.

So, your short goal will be, **"I will lose 10 pounds in 2 months"** which is more <u>attainable</u> then saying, **"I will lose 10 pounds in 1 week."**

Remember, the purpose of setting **<u>health and fitness goals</u>** is to assist you in achieving a healthy life, so you want to achieve lots of morale-boosting **smaller goals** first in order to work your way towards achieving your **major goals**.

4) SMA<u>R</u>T – 'R' stands for <u>Rewarding</u>

Make your goal <u>rewarding</u> and something that you can be <u>excited</u> about achieving.

For example, **"Losing 30 pounds by June 1^{st,} 2020 will help me to have an amazing beach body ready for the summer."**

5) SMAR<u>T</u> – 'T' stands for <u>Time-bound</u>

Set a <u>specific time</u> for completing and achieving your health goals.

In addition, don't stress yourself out if you don't **100%** achieve your goal.

For example, if your goal was to lose **30 pounds in 6 months** but you only lost **23 pounds in 6 months**, then be happy and excited about this great accomplishment.

Keep in mind that it's not a matter of whether or not you were able to complete your health goal **100%**.

Instead, what is important is that you achieved some **great results** and you stayed focused and committed to **achieving** your health and fitness goals and that is **ALL** that matters.

For more information about
Weight Loss and Health visit…
https://www.30daybellyfatloss.com/

Chapter 6 - <u>The Mind-Body Connection of a Healthy Diet</u>

Conversely, the **ill-effects** of an unbalanced diet are several and varied.

For example, having **low energy levels, as well as mood swings and feeling tired** all the time are just a few signs that your diet is **unhealthy and unbalanced**.

In addition, an **unhealthy and unbalanced diet** can cause problems with maintenance of body tissues, growth and development, brain and nervous system function, as well as problems with your bones and immune and digestive systems.

It is important to mention that when your body does not get a certain amount of **vitamins and nutrients** that it needs, you may suffer from **malnutrition.**

Symptoms of malnutrition include **lack of energy, irritability and a weak immune system** which can lead to frequent colds or allergies.

In addition, when you suffer from malnutrition, your body suffers from **mineral and vitamin depletion** which can trigger a variety of health concerns including anemia.

As stated before, since **the body is all connected** (your brain, your immune system, your emotions, etc.,) you will come to realize that having an **unhealthy body** will result in an unhealthy feelings and emotions which can even lead to depression.

Therefore, consider that when you **nourish** your body with these **amazing superfoods** and complement them with other **nutrient-dense and healthy fresh foods**, your spirit and overall wellbeing will be **vitalized and healthy** as a result of eating these powerful superfoods.

It is important to state that many modern diets based on prepackaged and processed convenience foods are most definitely lacking in many vitamins and minerals, which can affect your mental capacities as well and cause irritability, confusion, and the feeling of 'being in a fog' all the time.

Therefore, consider that **superfoods** can be the basis of a sound, healthy, nutritious **solution** to curing many of the **illnesses, sicknesses and diseases** that a person may encounter as a result of not eating a healthy diet.

<u>Color Your Way to Daily Health</u>

It's important that you eat plenty of different fruits and vegetables every day.

Diets rich in fruits and vegetables can **help to reduce** the risk of cancer and other chronic diseases.

In addition, fruits and vegetables provide essential vitamins and minerals, fiber, and other nutrients that are important for good health.

It is also important to state that most fruits and vegetables are naturally **low in fat and calories** and are also quite filling.

There is a fruit and vegetable health program called the **5 A Day for Better Health** program.

The **5 A Day for Better Health** program focuses on getting you to eat a combination of **5 servings** of fruits and vegetables every day.

The **5 A Day for Better Health** program provides easy ways to add more fruits and vegetables into your **daily eating habits** by using them as snacks, desserts and with salads or soups or even drinking them as **smoothies**.

It is very important to try to **eat a wide variety** of colorful (orange, yellow, red, green, white, blue and purple) vegetables and fruits every day.

By eating vegetables and fruit from each color group, you will benefit from the essential **vitamins, minerals, and fiber** that each color group has to offer alone and in combination.

There's several different, yet simple ways to start incorporating more vegetables and fruits into your familiar and favorite meals.

You can begin your mornings by drinking **100 percent fruit or vegetable juice**.

You can also slice bananas or strawberries and add them on top of your oatmeal.

You can also have a salad with your lunch and an apple for an afternoon snack.

You can also experiment with **blending** fruits and vegetables together in a blender to make super delicious and healthy **smoothies**.

Also, try to always include some **vegetables** with your dinner and consider making fruit a **dessert** after dinner.

Don't be afraid to try new fruits and vegetables in order to increase your vegetable and fruit intake. Also consider that there are so many choices when selecting fruits and vegetables.

You never know…kiwis, asparagus, and mangos may become your new **favorite foods**.

Therefore, keep your meals fresh and interesting by combining fruits and vegetables of different flavors and colors, like red grapes with pineapple chunks, or cucumbers and red peppers.

Also, get in the habit of keeping fruits and vegetables visible and easily accessible – you'll tend to eat them more often if they are easily accessible.

<u>Healthy Eating "Cheat Sheet"</u>

Healthy eating can be tough, even for the most disciplined person.

In addition, there are so many **temptations** in the world and all around us that sometimes it can seem like there is nothing we can do to make healthy choices.

Utilizing the knowledge in this **Cheat Sheet** will help you to make better **choices** about the foods that you eat.

In addition, you will also learn how the foods you eat **affect your body** so you will be more aware of why it is so important to make good food choices when it is time to eat.

<u>Why Eat Healthy?</u>

1) The standard American diet is dangerous. It is called the **SAD diet** for a reason, as processed foods are carcinogenic and unsustainable.

2) Eating junk food makes you susceptible to **disease**.

3) Other medical issues can also become problematic, like high blood pressure and diabetes.

<u>Understanding Your Relationship with Food</u>

1) Observe and be honest about your **eating habits**.

2) If you don't believe there is hope for the future it is hard to have the **motivation** to set and achieve health and fitness goals.

3) Evaluate your sense of **self-discipline** when it comes to eating and determine where you struggle so that you can begin to address the issue.

<u>The Dangers of Diet Trends</u>

1) Designed to make people **money**, not help people lose weight and maintain weight loss.

2) Often physically dangerous and sometimes lethal.

3) Makes you gain more weight in the long run by ruining your metabolism.

<u>How Food Can Be Your Medicine</u>

1) Consider the ancient healing art of **<u>Ayurveda</u>** which promotes **good health** and is based on whole natural foods similar to the Mediterranean diet.

2) Healthy foods **strengthen** the body and **protect** against disease.

3) Vitamin C can help **heal** the body actively.

4) Vegetables and Fruits provide important **antioxidants, vitamins and nutrients** for the body.

5) Healthy foods can **improve** your skin, beauty and overall health.

6) Eliminates **toxins** from the body.

7) Aids in **weight loss**.

8) **Heals** the body and **prevents** disease.

The Best Meat to Eat for Healthy Living

1) Grass-fed beef
2) Organic chicken
3) Organic turkey
4) Ethically raised fish

The Dangers of Processed Foods

1) Cause long-term medical problems
2) Excessive amounts of sugar, salt and fat
3) Carcinogenic chemicals
4) Low in **fiber** so you consume more food but burn fewer calories

Meal Planning

1) **Visualize** a healthy future.
2) Take time to seek out new recipes to try and experiment with.

3) **Organize** your recipes in a notebook, folder or binder.

4) Use **programs and apps** to help you create meal plans.

5) Stick with your meal plans to form **good habits**.

For more information about

Weight Loss and Health visit…

https://www.30daybellyfatloss.com/

Chapter 7 - <u>21 Days to a Healthier Heart (Challenge)</u>

21 Days to a Healthier Heart is about making smarter **food choices** and not feeling miserable or deprived.

Plain and simple, **YOU** are in control of your health.

In addition, it's easier than you think to start living a **heart-healthy lifestyle**.

Use the following strategies below to improve your **Health and your Heart in 21 Days**.

<u>Week 1-Getting Started</u>

Day 1 - Know your numbers.

You need to know your key **health numbers** in relation to your **heart health** in order to be able to track your progress.

If you have not been to a doctor in the last 3 months, make an appointment.

If you have, then get your blood test results.

Your doctor will test you for a range of things, but the most important in relation to the health of your **heart** are:

- blood pressure
- weight and height
- blood glucose reading
- total cholesterol
- LDL cholesterol
- HDL cholesterol
- triglycerides

Day 2 - Start from Where You Are

Once you know your numbers, start a **health journal** which requires you to **write down** the most important details of your health. Remember to be **honest** with yourself!

Day 3 - Set Health Goals

Once you know where you are, you can **set goals** for where you wish to go in terms of your heart health.

Choose **one goal**, like lowering cholesterol or losing weight and go for it.

Days 4 to 7 – Habits

Once you know your numbers and you set your goals, you can start making easy **heart-healthy changes** in terms of <u>eating habits, physical activity, and making smarter food choices</u>.

<u>Week 2 - Progressing</u>

Now that you have a much better idea about your **heart health**, it is time to add more healthy **strategies** and continue to **track** your progress.

Day 8 - Choose an Eating Lifestyle

There are many heart healthy choices but the **Mediterranean Diet** is the one diet that is **easy to follow** and that will keep you healthy.

Therefore, prepare yourself for indulging in the Mediterranean Diet by purchasing the **necessary foods** that are required for you to eat.

Day 9 - Learn More About Healthy Fats

When it comes to eating **healthy fats**, make sure to include the following foods:

- Extra Virgin Olive Oil

- Avocados
- Unsalted nuts (walnuts, almonds, Brazilian nuts, etc.,)
- Flaxseeds, Chia seeds, pumpkin seeds,
- Fatty fish such as salmon, tuna and sardines

Day 10 - Eat More Fresh Fruits and Veggies

There are many **heart healthy choices**, so the easiest way to remember is to try to eat a **rainbow** of fruits and vegetables every day.

In addition, consider that fruits and veggies are very **versatile**, so they can be eaten for breakfast, lunch and dinner and they can also be used in **smoothies and as desserts**.

Days 11 to 14

You've been progressing well. For the rest of the week you will continue to make **easy** heart healthy changes and track your progress.

Week 3 - Making More Heart-Healthy Changes

You're doing great. Now it's time to add more **healthy strategies** and continue to track your progress.

Day 15 - Get Fond of Fish

Eating **fatty fish** is important because it contains many **heart-healthy nutrients**, lowers your rate of heart attacks and strokes, keeps your brain functioning at optimal levels and prevents and treats depression.

Some good heart-healthy choices of fatty fish include **Salmon, Tuna, Sardines, Herring, Mackerel, and Cod.**

Day 16 - Go Nuts for Nuts

While it is true that nuts can be high in fat, they are also **filling** and contain many heart-healthy **nutrients**, antioxidants, help with weight loss and contain fiber.

However, keep in mind that you want to make sure you eat **Unsalted Nuts** such as walnuts, almonds, pistachios, cashews and pecans.

Day 17 - Dealing with Stress

Stress can have serious negative effects on your heart's health.

More specifically, stress causes a lot of **wear and tear** on the heart's blood vessels.

In addition, <u>**severe stress**</u> can even lead to **cardiovascular disease**.

However, consider that eating a lot of **healthy foods** greatly <u>reduces</u> stress.

For example:
1) Although not a food but **Tea** helps to reduce stress.

2) Dark Chocolate has **antioxidants** that reduces stress.

3) **Whole grain foods** reduce stress and improve your mood.

4) Avocados have **omega-3's** that help to reduce stress.

5) Fatty fish such as **tuna, salmon, sardines and mackerel** fight off stress.

6) Healthy, unsalted nuts such as **walnuts, almonds and cashews** help to reduce stress.

7) **Citrus fruits and strawberries** greatly help to reduce stress.

As you can see, there are many **healthy and powerful foods** that you can eat in order to reduce stress, keep you calm and improve your mood.

Days 18 to 21 – Your Heart is Interconnected
This week you have made **great changes** for improving your heart's health.

In addition, you will also be looking at your heart's health **holistically or interconnected** to the rest of your body.

So, this means that your heart is **interconnected** to your body, your mind, your emotions and your spirit.

So basically, the **foods that you eat** and the **health of your heart** is going to affect your entire **body, mind, emotions and spirit**.

So, if you have a **healthy heart** then you will also have a healthy body, mind, spirit and healthy thoughts.

Now consider that not only has your **heart improved**, but so has your body, your mind and your spirit.

Simply see the health of your heart, the health of your body, the health of your mind and the health of your spirit as **'holistic' or interconnected**.

Therefore, when the health of your **heart** improves, your overall **health** improves.

The **21 Days to a Healthier Heart Challenge** may be over but you have laid the foundations for a new heart-healthy lifestyle that can lower your risk of heart attacks and strokes and that offers a wide number of health benefits such as fighting off high blood pressure and Type 2 diabetes.

<u>How Food Can Be Your Medicine</u>

The same way that not eating healthy can make you **sick** is the same way that eating healthy foods can often times **cure** you of **illness** and provide you with **relief** when you are suffering.

Actually, eating healthy foods can also act as a **preventative measure** to take against illness.

In fact, there is an entire method of **healing** around India for thousands of years called **Aryuveda**.

This ancient **healing style** is utilized in order to treat any **illness** a person has by simply changing a person's **diet**.

Therefore, consider that food is literally the **medicine** that has helped to keep the people of India alive for centuries.

And, this idea of using **food as medicine** for curing illnesses can still be applicable today.

In fact, many **remedies for illnesses** are simply healthy foods that have **anti-inflammatory properties** as well as the ability to **nourish** your body from the inside out.

Something to think about is that **everything** from infection to cancer has been known to be impacted by **healthy eating choices**.

And with this ancient healing art of **Aryuveda** along with the **Mediterranean diet**, healthy eating truly impacts the health of people.

Of course, a lot of modern technology will frown upon these methods because they have not been scientifically investigated, but a lot of it has been tried and true for thousands of years and will continue to impact the body.

Whether you believe that **food is medicine** or not, the fact remains that food can ultimately determine whether or not you are susceptible to **illness**.

Simply, if you eat well, your body will be **stronger** and it will be able to fight off **illnesses and diseases** far easier than if you were **malnourished** eating unhealthy foods.

Something to keep in mind is that without the proper **vitamins and minerals** in your body, it can be almost impossible to fight off the negative effects of illness.

If you are eating **unhealthy unprocessed foods**, certain types of these foods can actually lead to **illnesses** and make you more susceptible to certain types of **cancer**.

Although cancer is still being researched and has not fully been understood by the scientific community well enough how to actually cure it, there are many instances of people who were able to live **long and healthy lives** simply by changing their diet and the foods they eat.

Healthy eating can help in decreasing the symptoms of many difficult and impossible to cure **diseases**, such as multiple sclerosis.

As long as you are making sure that everything that you put into your body is **nourishing** and is providing your organs and cells with all of the fuel and resources that they need in order to keep your body strong, they will continue to do that.

However, if you are actively sabotaging your body by eating **unhealthy processed foods**, then your immune system will not be able to defend your body from sickness, illnesses and disease.

That is why it is so important for you to take heed of the way you are nourishing your body.

If you are not making active and conscientious choices about the foods that you eat, you could be setting yourself up for **failure** in ways that you may live to **regret**.

<u>Setting a Healthy Example</u>

When you've taken all the right steps to intentionally **change your diet, improve your health, and transform your body** for the better, you'll be able to deal with any hurdles and setbacks that you encounter in life with a much calmer mind.

Come to realize that it is requires making a **strong commitment** for succeeding at living a **healthy lifestyle**.

Therefore, make a commitment to make the **Mediterranean diet** part of your new healthy lifestyle.

In addition, always have an **abundance** of foods from the **Mediterranean diet food list** available so that you can make sure you succeed with the Mediterranean diet.

You also want to make sure that you **enjoy the process** of living a healthy lifestyle along your journey to a healthier you.

Remember, your **decision** to improve your health and all of your effort and enthusiasm to live a **healthier life** will pay off in your own life as well as affect everyone you come in contact with.

In addition, family members, friends, loved ones, acquaintances, and casual contacts will be **influenced** by your dedication and genuine interest in improving your health and your life.

With a renewed **perspective** on health living and an obvious growth of **knowledge** on the Mediterranean diet you will be someone that can offer **guidance and compassion** to others from your own experience.

Being a good **role model** for those special people in your life can be **motivation** enough to stick with the battle of improving your health.

While you'll start out on the path to **improving your health** with many questions, possible frustrations and an air of uncertainty, you can feel confident that those thoughts will soon pass and you will become a **leader** of healthy living.

Simply spread the **Happiness** of **Healthy Living** with every person you come in contact.

And if you are ever confronted with self-doubt along your journey to a **healthier** life then read the following quote as inspiration:

"Never underestimate the power of a small group of committed people to change the world. In fact, it is the only thing that ever has." ~**Margaret Mead**

Remember, through your **individual choice** to be healthier, whatever your underlying reasons are, you could be quite a **role model** to many people around you.

Hopefully your positive example of **healthy living** will rub off and start a chain reaction – a **paradigm shift** – which helps people to make better **food choices** and **educates** people that healthy living is truly important for living a great life.

For more information about

Weight Loss and Health visit…

https://www.30daybellyfatloss.com/

Chapter 8 – <u>Mediterranean Superfoods: You Are What You Eat</u>

Recent dietary research has uncovered **14 different nutrient-dense foods** that time and time again promote good overall health.

These nutrient-dense healthy foods are many times referred to as **"superfoods."**

In addition, these "superfoods" tend to have fewer calories than other foods as well as higher levels of vitamins and minerals than other foods.

Another important thing to mention about these "superfoods" is that they also contain many **disease-fighting antioxidants** which prevent us from various illnesses and diseases.

Consider that foods such as beans (legumes), berries (especially blueberries), broccoli, green tea, nuts (especially walnuts), oranges, pumpkin, salmon, soy, spinach, tomatoes, whole grains and oats and yogurt can all help stop and even reverse diseases such as **hypertension, diabetes, Alzheimer's Disease and some forms of cancer.**

And where one kind of superfood might have an effect on a certain part of the body, it can also have a positive effect on the health of other **body functions and performance**, since the whole body (from the inside) is connected.

For example, eating blueberries will **improve your mood** and if you are feeling great you are likelier to want to exercise and get a great workout.

Another example is dark chocolate. Dark chocolate increases your energy levels and greatly improves your mood.

So, if your energy levels are high and you are feeling great, you are going to want to do more and achieve more, and simply feel all around great about yourself.

By making these **14 superfoods** part of your daily diet plan, you won't need any silly weight loss gimmicks or fly-by-night weight loss programs because these **superfoods** are sure to get you (and keep you) lean, fit and healthy.

<u>Superfoods</u>

We always hear about the many wonderful foods that are good to eat, and good for us.

More specifically, we always hear about eating fruits, vegetables and healthy nuts.

However, there are a wide variety of fruits, vegetables and different kinds of nuts to eat.

Therefore, wouldn't it be simpler to have a few **superfoods** that you can always refer to and eat in order to be **super healthy, fit and lean**?

To help you in your endeavors of living a **healthy lifestyle and a healthy life** you can use the list compiled below as a quick reference list of **9 superfoods** that will help you to **lose weight, look younger and feel great.**

In addition, some additional foods will be added as a way to give you more options in order to improve your healthy living lifestyle.

Also, keep in mind that these superfoods are not listed in any specific order according to nutritional value.

Super Foods For Weight loss, More Energy and Longevity

#1 Apples

Apples are a great superfood for many reasons including the ability to reduce the risk of heart disease, fight off certain cancers, reduce high blood pressure, and prevent type-2 diabetes.

Apples are also great because they improve your respiratory system by preventing lung cancer and asthma.

By consuming apples on a daily basis, your body gets fiber, potassium and antioxidants, such as Vitamin C and polyphenols.

Studies show that the real benefit of eating apples comes from all the combined nutrients and vitamins apples have (fiber, potassium and antioxidants such as Vitamin C and polyphenols).

To get the most out of eating apples for improving your health, eat a wide variety of apples and make sure that you eat the peel, which contains several times more antioxidants than the inside of an apple.

Remember, the old saying, **"An apple a day keeps the doctor away."**

#2 Avocados

Avocados are a powerful superfood that have become very popular in the past few years as a result of its health benefits.

For example, avocados contain important nutrients such as Vitamin K, Folate, Vitamin C, Potassium, and Vitamin B5 to name a few.

Avocados do not contain any cholesterol or sodium and are very low in saturated fat.

Avocados also have fiber which helps to keep your weight down because they help you to feel full, which triggers your body to stop eating.

Avocados may also reduce arthritis and prevent cancer.

#3 Dark Chocolate

When you want to indulge a little bit with your healthy eating habits, you can help yourself to some dark chocolate.

Dark chocolate has some great health benefits. For example, dark chocolate contains lots of polyphenols which are **plant compounds** that provide a lot of health benefits.

For example, these **plant compounds** found in dark chocolate improve digestion and brain health, protect against heart disease, type 2 diabetes and certain cancers.

Dark chocolate is also considered to be a **natural anti-inflammatory food** which is another benefit of eating dark chocolate.

In 2000, a study published by the American Journal of Clinical Nutrition showed that the effect on blood flow from **high flavanol cocoa** found in dark chocolate was similar to taking a low-dose aspirin.

This means that dark chocolate could possibly be used to treat ailments like **minor pains, aches or headaches.**

Here are some other benefits of eating dark chocolate:

1) Improves your brain function.

2) Provides antioxidants which help you to look younger.

3) Improves your blood flow and prevents blood clots.

4) Reduces stress, improves your mood, relaxes you and generally makes you feel better.

To get the most benefits of eating dark chocolate, aim to eat dark cholate that is made of at least **85% cocoa beans**.

#4 Extra Virgin Olive Oil

There has been much discussion lately about the benefits of the **Mediterranean diet**.

Well Extra Virgin Olive oil is one of the **main components** of the Mediterranean diet and its benefits are outstanding.

Olive oil is a great **substitute** for other oils and fats and has been shown to reduce the risk of breast cancer as well as colon cancer.

In addition, olive oil also lowers blood pressure and improves the health of your cardiovascular system.

Here are some other benefits of Extra Virgin Olive Oil:

1) Contains antioxidants which help prevent chronic diseases.
2) Contains nutrients that fight inflammation in the body.
3) Helps to reduce and prevent strokes.
4) Fights off Alzheimer's Disease and prevents diabetes.

For best results use **extra virgin olive oil** that is cold pressed and greenish in color.

#5 Garlic

Another important food component of the Mediterranean diet is **garlic** which is great for improving your cardiovascular system.

By eating garlic regularly, you can reduce your blood pressure, triglyceride levels (a type of fat found in your blood) and your LDL (bad) cholesterol.

Garlic is also known to have **anti-inflammatory agents and antibiotic properties** which reduce inflammation in the body and fight off bacteria in the body.

Here are some other benefits of garlic:

1) Contains vitamin C, vitamin B6, manganese and other important vitamins required for the body.

2) Improves your immune system and helps prevent the flu and common cold.

3) Reduces blood pressure and increases bone health.

4) Improves your cholesterol levels and reduces heart disease.

5) Has antioxidants that prevent Alzheimer's Disease and Dementia.

6) Helps you to live longer and improves longevity.

7) Improves physical performance.

To get all the health benefits of garlic, try to eat garlic a few times a week.

Raw garlic is best, but cooked is also good.

Keep in mind that dried garlic and garlic supplements don't have the same benefits as fresh garlic.

#6 Raw Honey

Honey is not often seen on many lists of healthy foods, but don't let that fool you.

Eating honey daily increases the amounts of **powerful antioxidants** your needs, prevents constipation, and reduces cholesterol and blood pressure.

Here are some other benefits of eating raw honey:

1) Improves your memory.
2) Reduces the risk of heart attacks, strokes and some types of cancer.
3) Increase blood flow to your heart and reduces the risk of blood clot formation.
4) Improves physical, athletic performance.

If you are running low on energy, reach for raw honey, not sugar.

Honey does a better job of maintaining blood sugar and increasing and maintaining your energy levels than any other sweeteners.

In addition, choose **dark honeys** over light ones, because dark honeys are higher in antioxidants and flavor.

Consuming one to two teaspoons of raw honey several times a week should help you get all the benefits raw honey has to offer.

#7 Kiwis

If you want to consume extreme quantities of **Vitamin C and Vitamin E** then start eating kiwis.

Kiwis are a powerful fruit that reduces the risk of **asthma, osteoarthritis, and colon cancer**.

In addition, kiwis are also known to **boost your immune system**, aid with digestion and reduce blood pressure and blood clotting.

An interesting point to keep in mind is that dietary **Vitamin E** appears to lower the risk of Alzheimer's Disease and by consuming kiwis, you get large amounts of Vitamin E without the calories that most other Vitamin E rich foods contain like nuts and oils.

Another important ingredient found in kiwis is lutein, which protects your eyes from the loss of vision.

To get all the health benefits that kiwis have to offer, try to consume a kiwi two to three times a week.

#8 Onions

Onions have some of the **same health benefits** as garlic because they are part of the same family.

Onions are known to be full of important vitamins and minerals such as Vitamin C, B Vitamins including folate (B9) and Potassium.

Onions also contain powerful **antioxidants and compounds** that fight inflammation, reduce high blood pressure and your cholesterol levels and protect you from blood clots.

Here are some other benefits of eating onions:

1) Protects you from cancer, diabetes and heart disease.
2) Improves your bone health.
3) Are rich in fiber and prebiotics which improves your digestive system.

Try to eat dishes containing onions at least three times a week, and make sure that you let the onions sit for 5 to 10 minutes after you cut them open.

If you are cooking onions and apply heat too soon to them, you will remove some of the health benefits that onions have to offer.

Also keep in mind that the more pungent the onions are, the better and healthier they are for you.

#9 Pomegranates

Pomegranates are considered to be one of the **healthiest fruits** in the world because they have so many health benefits.

For example, pomegranates are full of amazing nutrients such as fiber, protein, Vitamin C, Folate, Vitamin K and Potassium.

Pomegranates are also a powerful **anti-inflammatory food**. As a result, pomegranates help to reduce chronic inflammation in the body.

Here are some other benefits of eating pomegranates:
1) Helps fight off prostate and breast cancer.
2) Lowers your blood pressure.
3) Fights off arthritis and joint pain.
4) Reduces the risk of heart disease.
5) Helps improve your memory and exercise performance.

As stated before, pomegranates are a powerful fruit and should be eaten as often as possible.

One thing to keep in mind is to stay away from pomegranate juices with added sugar.

11 Super Foods That Keep You Healthy

Get ready to experience a volume of information on some of the **healthiest foods** in the world.

Here is a list of the **Top 11 superfoods** that most health experts agree on.

You should tell everyone you know about these superfoods and enjoy them at your next meal.

From fruits and vegetables, to whole grains, nuts, beans and legumes.

This power-packed nutritional inventory will take you into the best years of your life and beyond.

Fruits

#1 Cantaloupe

Just eating a quarter of cantaloupe provides almost all the **vitamin A** needed in one day.

Vitamin A is important because it provides **antioxidants** that destroy cancerous cells.

In addition, Vitamin A is an important nutrient for your **eyes**. Vitamin A also strengthens your teeth and bones.

Since the beta-carotene in a cantaloupe converts to vitamin A, you get both nutrients, beta-carotene and Vitamin A at once.

Like an orange, cantaloupe is also an excellent source of vitamin C, which helps improve your immune system.

Cantaloupes are also a good source of vitamin B6, dietary fiber, folate, niacin, and potassium, which help maintain good blood sugar levels and keep your metabolism working properly.

One last thing to mention about cantaloupe is that this powerful fruit may help reduce your risk of heart disease, stroke, and cancer.

#2 Blueberries

These mildly sweet and sometimes tangy berries are so powerful that they help to **fight off cancer**.

Blueberries are low in calories and provide **powerful antioxidants** which enhance the effects of vitamin C.

In addition, these antioxidants found in blueberries help prevent cataracts, glaucoma, hemorrhoids, peptic ulcers and heart disease.

#3 Tomatoes

Although many people think tomatoes are a vegetable, they are actually a fruit.

Tomatoes are great because they fight off heart disease and certain cancers such as prostate cancer, breast cancer, lung cancer and cancer of the pancreas.

Tomatoes are also good sources of vitamin C, A, and K.

In a 2004 study, it was found that tomato juice alone can help reduce blood clotting.

Fresh, organic tomatoes deliver three times as much of the cancer-fighting antioxidant lycopene then regular tomatoes.

Even organic ketchup is better for you than regular ketchup!

Look for tomato paste and sauces that contain the whole tomato (including peels) because you will absorb 75% more of the antioxidant lycopene and almost two times the amount of beta-carotene then regular tomato paste and sauce.

Vegetables

#4 Sweet Potatoes

As an excellent source of vitamin, A, C, and manganese, sweet potatoes are also a good source of copper, dietary fiber, vitamin B6, potassium and iron.

Those individuals who are smokers or prone to second-hand smoke may benefit greatly from eating sweet potatoes because they help protect against emphysema.

For a unique but healthy dessert, cut a cooked sweet potato into cubes and add slices of banana on top it.

Then lightly pour maple syrup over the top and add a dash or two of cinnamon. Add chopped walnuts for an even healthier kick.

#5 Spinach and Kale

A **cancer-fighter and cardio-helper,** spinach and kale top the list as far as some of the best green leafy vegetables to eat.

Much like broccoli, both kale and spinach provide an excellent source of vitamin A and C.

Kale is surprisingly a good source of calcium at 25% per cup.

Vitamin K, which helps reduce bone loss, is also abundantly found in spinach providing almost 200% of the recommended daily intake.

Whole Grains

#6 Whole Grain Bread, Pasta and Brown Rice

There are many people that say whole grains are not healthy but it all depends on what kind of whole grains you are talking about.

Whether it's bread or pasta, the first thing to check for when purchasing whole grain bread and pasta is to make sure it is **100% whole grain**.

Remember to check the list of ingredients on the package. For example, look for the exact phrase **"whole wheat flour"** as one of the first ingredients listed in whole wheat bread.

If it's not listed as such, then it's not whole grain.

Keep in mind that **wheat bran** is a cancer-fighting grain that helps us to regulate our bowel movements.

Brown rice is also a better choice than refined grain (white rice) for the same reason as choosing whole wheat bread.

Whole wheat flour or brown rice that turns into **white flour** or **white rice** actually destroys between 50-90% of vitamin B3, vitamin B1, vitamin B6, manganese, phosphorus, iron, and all of the dietary fiber and essential fatty acids we need.

Even when processed white flour or white rice is "enriched," it is not in the same form as the original unprocessed kind.

In fact, 11 nutrients are actually lost and are not replaced during the "enrichment" process!

Therefore, make sure to always look at the ingredients carefully when buying **Whole Grain Bread, Pasta or Brown Rice.**

<u>Nuts</u>

#7 Walnuts

Walnuts are packed with **omega-3 fats**, which is considered a "good" healthy fat.

A quarter cup of walnuts would take care of about 90% of the omega-3s needed in one day.

Walnuts provide many health benefits including cardiovascular protection, better cognitive function, anti-inflammatory advantages relating to asthma, rheumatoid arthritis, and inflammatory skin diseases like eczema and psoriasis.

Walnuts can even help against cancer and also support the immune system.

Therefore, consider adding a handful of walnuts to your diet.

Beans and Legumes

#8 Black Beans and Lentils

While black beans are a good source of fiber that can lower cholesterol, so are lentils.

The high fiber content in both black beans and lentils helps to maintain your blood sugar levels.

In addition, black beans and lentils are also considered to be **fat-free** and a good source of **high-quality protein** with B-vitamins and additional minerals.

Because of the high fiber content found in black beans and lentils, they will help to keep you filling full and they will also help you to lose weight.

If possible, try to eat a variety of beans and lentils such as pinto and kidney beans to get the most nutrients as possible.

Also, consider making a delicious soup using beans and lentils with the addition of tomatoes, onions, garlic and your favorite spices for a super delicious, healthy meal.

<u>Dairy</u>

#9 Almond Milk and Yogurt

Almond milk, which is made of almonds, contains important nutrients such as Vitamins E and D, potassium, calcium, protein and magnesium.

Almond milk has no cholesterol and it reduces bad cholesterol in the body.

In addition, almond milk helps to keep your bones strong and helps to reduce blood pressure.

Another thing that makes almond milk so great is that it helps to fight off cancer, boosts your immune system, it is good for your digestive system and it improves the functioning of your brain.

Now believe it or not but yogurt has been consumed by people for **hundreds of years**.

Eating **good plain, unprocessed yogurt** offers the best health benefits a person needs

For example, yogurt has been found to reduce the risk of heart disease, osteoporosis and helps with controlling your weight.

Yogurt also includes essential nutrients such as phosphorous, vitamin B2, vitamin B12, vitamin B5, zinc, potassium, and protein.

Yogurt is also good for your digestive system and strengthens your immune system.

Just remember to always eat plain, unprocessed yogurt.

Seafood

#10 Salmon

Salmon is a heart-healthy food and is recommended to eat at least twice a week.

Salmon is high in protein, low in saturated fat and high in omega-3 fats (the essential fatty acids that are also found in those walnuts mentioned earlier).

More specifically, salmon reduces inflammation, lowers blood pressure and decreases risk factors for disease.

In addition, salmon contains important B vitamins which protect your heart and brain.

When choosing salmon, it's best to stay away from farm raised salmon and instead select wild caught salmon.

#11 Green Tea

Although not a food per say, the powerful health benefits of green tea are worth mentioning.

Green tea is full of **antioxidants and nutrients** that improve brain function, reduce your risk of cancer and help with weight loss.

In addition, green tea protects your brain from Alzheimer's Disease as well as Parkinson's Disease.

Green tea has been known to even reduce your risk of diabetes as well as cardiovascular disease.

Developing the habit of drinking green tea on a daily basis is quite easy to do.

Simply go to the supermarket and choose from one of the many kinds of green tea that are available.

For more information about

Weight Loss and Health visit…

https://www.30daybellyfatloss.com/

Chapter 9 - <u>What to Do Next</u>

Now that you know what superfoods are important for your health, make a commitment to eating them on a daily basis.

In addition, realize that by eating these superfoods on a daily basis you are investing in your health.

You are also saving money by eating these superfoods because these superfoods will keep you lean, healthy and fit and this means you will spend less money on going to the doctor and pay less on medical bills.

<u>Superfoods for Super Skin</u>

It's been said that **"we are what we eat,"** and that sentiment definitely holds true when it comes to our skin.

Our skin is our body's biggest organ and it deserves all the nutritional care we can give it.

So, take a look at what you've been feeding yourself and consider that what you eat not only affects your **body and brain but also your skin**.

It is important to state that one of the most important components of skin health is vitamin A and probably some of the best food sources of vitamin A are:

- Salmon
- Hard-boiled eggs
- Sweet potatoes
- Kale and Spinach
- Carrots
- Mangos

As stated before, the health of our skin depends on Vitamin A.

As a result, it is important to make sure you're eating foods rich in **antioxidants** such as blackberries, blueberries, strawberries, and plums.

The benefits of eating foods rich in antioxidants for healthier skin are plentiful.

In addition, the antioxidants and other important compounds found in plant-based foods are essential for **protecting your skin from damage**.

It is also important to state that, foods high in vitamin A protect the skin against **premature aging** and keeps the skin looking younger.

Other important foods that are high in antioxidants which are great for your skin are chia seeds, oats, turmeric, olive oil and green tea.

Essential fatty acids (EFAs) or "healthy fats" are also essential for your skin because they keep your skin healthy and allow nutrients to provide you with more youthful looking skin.

Therefore, include eating **salmon, walnuts and flaxseeds** as part of your diet because these foods contain an abundance of "healthy fats."

Keep in mind that eating good-quality healthy oils such as **Extra Virgin Olive Oil** helps to keep your skin **lubricated** and keeps it looking and feeling healthier.

To get the most health benefits from consuming Extra Virgin Olive Oil, all you really need is about one or two tablespoons a day.

Something you want to keep in mind is that eating processed and refined sugars can cause inflammation in your body which can lead to "skin breakouts" or **rashes**.

Therefore, you want to stay away from processed foods and refined sugars and instead try to eat more natural foods like fruits and vegetables.

Although not a food, drinking green tea has anti-inflammatory properties that helps prevent oily skin, acne, makes your skin look younger and it may even help reduce the risk of skin cancer.

Water also plays an important role in your overall health, and it has a profound effect on your skin's health as well.

Well-hydrated skin is healthy and young-looking. Water also "flushes out" and **removes toxins** out of your body so that the toxins have less chance to do damage to your body.

So, remember, to have healthier, more youthful looking skin, all you have to do is eat healthy foods high in Vitamin A.

By eating foods high in Vitamin A, your body, your brain and even your skin will be a lot healthier.

Below are **6 of the World's Top Anti-Aging Superfoods**:

1) Goji Berries

Goji berries are considered to be one of the most **nutritionally dense foods** on earth and contain a lot of vitamins, minerals, amino acids, antioxidants and essential fatty acids.

For example, goji berries contain 500 times more **vitamin C** than oranges and more beta-carotene than carrots making them a superb source of vitamin A.

In addition, goji berries are also known to contain more of the muscle building mineral **"iron"** than steak.

Goji berries also rank as having some of the **highest concentration of antioxidants** than any other foods.

Because of all of the high amounts of vitamins, minerals, amino acids, antioxidants and essential fatty acids that goji berries contain, it is no wonder that they are considered to be a powerful anti-aging food.

Originating in Tibet and greatly favored in **traditional medicine**, goji berries have many noted health benefits including boosting your immune system, lowering cholesterol, improving your vision, fighting cancer cells, reducing depression and aiding with weight loss.

Goji berries are also found to stimulate the secretion of **Human Growth Hormone (HGH),** a natural but powerful hormone that slows down the **aging process** and helps you to look and feel younger.

The most well documented case of **longevity** is that of Li Qing Yuen, who lived to the age of 252.

Born in 1678, he is said to have married 14 times with 11 generations of posterity before his death in 1930. Li Qing Yuen reportedly consumed goji berries daily.

A study cited in Dr. Mindell's book **'Goji: The Himalayan Health Secret,'** observed that 67 percent of **elderly people** that were given a daily dose of goji berries for 3 weeks experienced dramatic immune system enhancement and a significant increase with their energy levels, mood, and improved sleep patterns.

2) Aloe Vera Leaves

Forget Botox, eat **Aloe Vera Leaves** to get more youthful, beautiful, wrinkle-free skin.

Although most people apply Aloe Vera on their skin, Aloe Vera Leaves are **safe to eat**.

What makes Aloe Vera Leaves so great is that eating Aloe Vera Leaves increases **collagen production** in the body.

Collagen is the most **abundant** protein in the human body. In addition, collagen is one of the **major building blocks** of strong and healthy bones, skin, muscles, tendons and ligaments.

The inner gel of the Aloe Vera Leaf contains around 200 active compounds with over **75 nutrients**. These nutrients include 20 minerals, 18 amino acids and 12 vitamins.

Aloe Vera Leaves have **anti-microbial properties** which help to fight fungi and bacteria.

In addition, Aloe Vera Leaves help **to reduce** inflammation, relieve pain and help heal cuts and burns.

Aloe Vera Leaves can also help your digestive system to work better, strengthen your immune system, and be highly effective at **healing, moisturizing and rejuvenating** your skin.

Aloe Vera is best eaten **fresh** when possible (you can actually order large Aloe Vera Leaves which last a few weeks refrigerated).

To eat Aloe Vera Leaves, all you have to do is **cut** the leaf into small pieces and use a spoon to scrape out the inside gel of the leaf.

You can then add the gel to fruit or even use it to make a smoothie.

So, remember, if you want more **beautiful and healthier skin**, consider eating Aloe Vera Leaves.

Aloe Vera Leaves can most certainly be an alternative to Botox.

3) Avocados

Avocados are considered to be a **"superfruit"** which have become very popular in the past few years due to their amazing health benefits.

Eating avocados will help to make your **skin smooth and soft**.

In addition, avocados also contain **vitamin E** which is a powerful antioxidant that helps **nourish and protect your skin**.

Avocados are also full of healthy fats, fiber and other important nutrients such as Vitamin K, Potassium, Vitamin C and Folate.

Avocados can lower your cholesterol, reduce heart disease and even prevent cancer.

Last, avocados can help you to lose weight and may reduce symptoms of arthritis.

4) Chlorella

Chlorella is a **green freshwater algae**. You cannot actually eat chlorella because it is very hard for the body to digest it. However, you can take it as a **supplement**.

Chlorella is considered to be a **superfood** because of its many health benefits.

For example, chlorella contains protein, Vitamin B12, Iron and Vitamin C, Omega-3s, Fiber and other vitamins and minerals.

In addition, chlorella helps the body to **"detox"** by removing harmful compounds from the body.

Chlorella can also help keep your immune system stay **healthy and strong** by fighting off infections and chronic diseases.

As a result of having a healthier and stronger immune system your **lifespan increases** and you live longer and healthier.

As stated before, chlorella is jam-packed with vitamins, minerals, antioxidants, enzymes and amino acids, making it an incredibly **rejuvenating and health-promoting superfood**.

An alternative to chlorella is **Spirulina**, another kind of algae that offers a lot of health benefits similar to chlorella.

5) Bee Pollen

Bee pollen is so healthy and good for you that it is considered to be not only a powerful superfood but also **medicine**.

Bee pollen helps to relieve inflammation, strengthens your immune system, reduces stress and works as a **powerful antioxidant**.

Bee pollen is considered to contain **250 types of nutrients, vitamins and antioxidants** and it can be eaten with foods such as oatmeal, smoothies or yogurt.

Bee pollen is also known to help with weight loss, **increase your lifespan**, heal wounds on the skin as well **soften and moisturize your skin**.

Because bee pollen has such outstanding benefits to providing a person with **young and beautiful skin**, it has been used to successfully treat acne and other **skin conditions** and beautify a person's skin as well as help people get all of its **anti-aging benefits**.

Overall, bee pollen has been called a **'prefect food'** because it is so nutritionally complete.

6) Coconut Oil

Coconut oil is removed from a coconut's kernels and can be both **consumed** or used on your **skin** for getting certain health benefits.

For example, coconut oil contains **healthy fats** that help with burning fat, increases your energy levels, fights off Alzheimer's Disease and helps your brain to function better.

Coconut oil also helps to fight off heart disease and kill harmful bacteria, viruses and fungi in the body.

Coconut oil is also great for increasing the 'good' cholesterol in your body as well as lowering the 'bad' cholesterol in your body.

Coconut oil can also be applied on your skin for **beautifying and moisturizing** your skin.

Coconut oil contains antioxidants that **protect your skin** from the sun as well as your hair from getting damaged.

Coconut oil can also be used to treat wounds, burns and certain **skin conditions**.

And if all of these health benefits weren't enough, coconut oil also contains powerful antioxidants that help **slow down the aging process**.

It can be said that coconut oil is essential for anyone that wants to live longer, look and feel younger as well as be healthier.

<u>Superfoods for a Super Long Life</u>

Research shows that important plant compounds found in foods such as **broccoli, bok choy, kale, cauliflower and**

cabbage work to strengthen your body's immune system to protect it from cancer, cardiovascular disease and even premature aging.

Research also shows that people who eat more **fruits and vegetables** live longer than those people that don't as a result of all the nutrients, vitamins, minerals and antioxidants they contain.

There is actually a group of people that live in Okinawa, Japan called, **Okinawans**, that are said to have the world's **longest life expectancy** as a result of their diet.

The Okinawans are said to have **low rates** of heart disease and cancer as a result of eating lots of fruits and veggies.

In addition, the Okinawans eat large quantities of **sweet potatoes** and disregard the Japanese staple of rice.

What we can learn from the Okinawans is to simply eat healthier foods in order to increase our lifespan.

The Road to Longevity

With advancements in science and research, in the near future doctors will be able to tell their patients exactly what diseases and illnesses they might be genetically predisposed to early on in a person's life, so that a person can immediately make changes to his/her diet.

So, once a person knows what disease or illnesses, he is susceptible to, that person will be able to use food as his **medicine**.

In addition, a person will be able to know what foods to eat and which foods to avoid in order to prevent a chronic disease from occurring.

In the meantime, many foods have already been determined to teach us which foods **strengthen** our immune systems, **increase** our energy levels, and **slow down** the aging process.

For example, lycopene, a powerful antioxidant that makes tomatoes red, also appears to reduce the risk for cardiovascular disease, fights off some forms of cancers, and prevent the loss of one's eyesight.

Pink grapefruit, guava, red bell peppers, and watermelon are also rich in the antioxidant lycopene.

Research shows that eating at least two cups of orange fruits and vegetables a day like sweet potatoes, squash and carrots greatly increases a person's intake of beta-carotene.

Beta-carotene is an **antioxidant** which converts to vitamin A, which is essential for healthy skin and protecting your eyes, and which may also reduce the risk of some cancers, cardiovascular disease, and osteoporosis.

Lutein which is another important vitamin found in orange produce combined with the powerful antioxidant, lycopene, are said to help **reduce** the risk of vision loss and may protect the skin from sun damage and even reduce wrinkles as well.

Fruits like mangos and cantaloupes are also full of beta-carotene and are another good source of Vitamin A.

Now if there is one major change that you must make to your diet then that would be to eat more **dark green leafy vegetables**.

Dark green leafy vegetables have been shown to significantly reduce your risk for heart disease, prevent cancer, help with weight loss, keep your brain working properly and prevent high blood pressure.

Dietary guidelines advise to eat dark green leafy vegetables at every meal.

In addition, eating frozen or packaged dark green leafy vegetables are just as good as fresh.

One last important group of healthy fats that are essential to the body and brain are **omega-3's**.

The heart-healthy omega-3's have been shown to keep your brain sharp and prevent your brain from cognitive decline.

Omega-3's also help to fight depression and anxiety, prevent heart attacks and strokes, and reduces inflammation in the body.

Omega-3's simply have too many health benefits to name them all.

However, omega-3's should most definitely be made part of a healthy diet.

In addition, eating fatty fish like salmon, sardines and tuna will help you get all the omega-3's your body and brain needs.

Below are some 7 superfoods that you can eat for increasing you lifespan:

1) Fish

Eating oily fish such as **salmon and sardines** will most definitely increase your lifespan.

Oily fish contains powerful vitamins such as Vitamin A and D which **strengthen** your immune system.

Oily fish are also rich in **omega-3's** which help to reduce heart disease, lowers your fish of suffering a stroke and keeps your brain functioning properly and fight off Alzheimer's Disease.

2) Green Tea

Although green tea is not a food, it is a **powerful drink** that will greatly improve your cardiovascular health, strengthen your immune system and lower your cholesterol.

Green tea is also full of **powerful antioxidants** which can help lower your risk of **cancer**.

In addition, research shows that people that drink green tea on a daily basis **live longer** than people that don't.

3) Extra Virgin Olive Oil

Extra virgin olive oil is considered to be a **healthy fat** that is used especially with the Mediterranean Diet.

Extra virgin olive oil has **powerful antioxidants** that reduce inflammation in the body as well as reduces your risk of stroke and heart disease.

In addition, extra virgin olive oil can help lower your risk of diabetes, improve bone health, protects you from certain kinds of cancers and reduces the risk of Alzheimer's disease and dementia.

Research also shows that consuming extra virgin olive oil can help you to **live longer**.

4) Garlic

Garlic is a **powerful superfood** that has been used for **thousands of years** as a result of its powerful health and therapeutic benefits.

For example, garlic helps to combat certain kinds of cancer, lowers your cholesterol and reduces heart attacks and heart disease.

In addition, garlic is also considered to be a **powerful antibiotic** that fights against intestinal infections, protects your heart from diabetes and heart damage and lowers high blood pressure.

Overall, garlic is a powerful superfood that has been eaten throughout history by many people from various cultures as a result of having very powerful health benefits.

5) Cranberries

This little fruit is full of **vitamins and powerful antioxidants** that helps reduce inflammation in the body, strengthens your immune system, fights off cancer and decreases blood pressure.

Cranberries also contain phytonutrients which are natural chemicals found in plant foods that help prevent disease and keep the body working properly.

Cranberries also reduce the risk of heart disease, helps with weight loss and improves your levels of "good" cholesterol.

Research also shows that cranberries help promote **longevity.**

6) Coffee Beans

Coffee beans contain flavonoids which are **antioxidants** that help prevent chronic diseases like heart disease.

In addition, the antioxidants contained in coffee beans help prevent **cancer, diabetes and strokes**.

Coffee beans also help with weight loss, reduces inflammation in the body, protects the nervous system from injuries and also protects the brain from Alzheimer Disease, Parkinson's Disease and multiple sclerosis.

Coffee beans also help with increasing a **person's lifespan**.

<u>Superfoods that Eliminate Stress</u>

Life has a way of getting the best of us some days.

Whether it's working too many hours, shuffling your kids all over town for their activities, taking care of your household, or dealing with personal or family matters, **stress** can most definitely take its toll on you **physically, mentally, emotionally, and spiritually**.

But there are simple steps you can take to **combat stress**, starting with the foods that you eat.

For example, avoiding **caffeine and alcohol** is a good start when it comes to reducing stress in your life.

In addition, stimulants like **caffeine** and depressants like **alcohol** can both **zap your energy** and rob you of the fuel you need to successfully cope with stress.

Sugary foods should also be avoided as well, as they cause your **blood sugar and energy levels** to spike then dip rapidly, which causes stress to your body and mind.

However, there are several superfoods out there that provide you with the **energy and nutrition** your body needs to keep stress in check.

For example, **avocados and bananas** are both full of potassium which help to keep your blood pressure low.

Although not a food but a powerful drink, **Tea** helps to relax you as well as calms your nerves.

Leafy green veggies like **Swiss Chard and spinach** contain magnesium which helps to reduce cortisol, a **stress hormone** in the body.

Eating fatty fish such as **salmon, sardines and tuna** contain omega-3 fats which help to keep you calm and relaxed.

Crunchy foods like **carrots and celery** are good healthy snacks that help to reduce stress.

Healthy nuts such as **almonds, walnuts and pistachios** also help to improve your immune system, reduce stress and provide the body with important vitamins and minerals such as zinc.

The ever so popular, **Dark Chocolate** helps to reduce stress and also improves your mood.

Foods high in **folic acid**, also known as **Vitamin B8**, help to improve your mood.

For example, **asparagus, legumes, eggs and beets** all contain Vitamin B8 which helps to improve your mood.

Believe it or not, but even lean cuts of **grass-fed beef** can help reduce stress.

Grass-fed Beef has high levels of iron, zinc and B vitamins that help to reduce stress and improve your mood.

However, you want to only consume **grass-fed beef** once in a while and you also want to stick to eating lean cuts of beef.

Whole grain cereal is also considered to reduce stress. You can even use **almond milk** to eat your whole grain cereal.

Almond milk contains **Vitamin E** which protects the body against cancer, arthritis and diabetes.

Cottage cheese is another good source of food for fighting off stress.

To add some flavor to your cottage cheese you can eat it with **fruit** that is high in **Vitamin C** such as guavas, kiwis, strawberries and oranges.

Vitamin C helps to reduce chronic diseases, lowers blood pressure, strengthens your immune system and prevents Dementia.

For more information about
Weight Loss and Health visit…
https://www.30daybellyfatloss.com/

Conclusion

First, I want to thank you for making it to the end of this eBook.

You have taken the responsibility for improving your life by learning how to improve your health with the **Mediterranean diet,** the power of **superfoods** and with a well-developed **health plan**.

Actually, the Mediterranean diet combined with exercise will **bulletproof** your body from illnesses, sickness and diseases so consider making some form of **exercise** part of your health plan.

Now that you are more knowledgeable about the Mediterranean Diet, superfoods and improving your overall health, it is important to immediately begin to take **ACTION** towards achieving your health goals.

You can begin by experimenting with eating different kinds of **fruits and vegetables** on a daily basis.

Also be aware of which fruits and vegetables you like and which, for whatever reason, you don't like.

You also want to make sure you consume a variety of **Mediterranean superfoods,** whether it is Tea, sardines, blueberries or Dark Chocolate for the purpose of getting a variety of vitamins and nutrients.

Last, you want to make your **Mediterranean meals and snacks** delicious so experiment by combining different food groups in order to discover your favorite Mediterranean meals and snacks.

Also remember that making a **decision** to eat healthy and working to improve your health is a **lifestyle change**.

Actually, improving your health through proper **nutrition and exercise** requires good daily habits whether it is eating vegetables at every meal or eating one piece of fruit every day.

Nevertheless, make a commitment to improving your health and your life by simply eating more and more **Mediterranean superfoods** every day.

STOP!

Before you go, I have included a **Bonus Chapter** that begins on the following page.

Please continue reading…

Bonus Chapter- <u>5 Simple Ways To Lose Belly Fat In 30 Days Or Less</u>

#1 Sleep More

According to research, sleep is more important than **nutrition and exercise**.

Research also shows that the more you sleep the more **fat you burn** because your metabolism functions better when your body gets between **7-9 hours of sleep**.

Consider that a lack of sleep will develop **stress** in your body causing you to gain **weight**.

More specifically, a lack of sleep increases your **appetite** as a result of the body being stressed from a lack of sleep.

In addition, a lack of sleep will also affect your **mood, energy levels and overall performance**.

As you can see, you want to make sure you sleep as much as possible especially if you want to **burn belly fat** effectively.

Remember, sleep is extremely important for losing belly fat and for being **successful** in overall life because it will **repair your body and mind** from all the mental and physical stress you put it through each and every day.

Therefore, start making getting enough sleep a **priority** in your life.

#2 Avoid Overeating With "Portion Control"

Overeating can cause weight gain which can lead to belly fat.

However, you can **prevent excess weight gain** and belly fat, from overeating by practicing **"portion control."**

"Portion control" is simply reducing the amount of food you eat by eating smaller portions.

The best way to reduce the amount of food that you eat is by using a small **food scale**.

You can also consider using a **smaller bowl or plate** for reducing the amount of food you eat.

However, using a **food scale** for reducing the amount of food you eat is **100% more accurate** than using a small bowl or plate.

When it comes to "portion control" using a food scale, all you have to do is simply **weigh your food** before you eat it so that you will know **exactly** how much food you are consuming for each meal.

So, if you want to simply lose a **few extra pounds** all you have to do is simply reduce the amount of food you are eating by using your food scale.

The concept of "portion control" is very popular with **bodybuilders, weightlifters and competitive athletes** because these individuals knows that a food scale helps them to lose weight or simply maintain their weight.

Nutritionists also advise people that suffer from **obesity** to also use a food scale to help them with losing weight.

So, if you think about it if "portion control" works for these individuals it will most definitely work for you.

#3 Practice Intermittent Fasting

Intermittent fasting is an **amazing and effective** way of quickly burning off belly fat.

Intermittent fasting is simply a **healthy eating method** and more of a **lifestyle** that any person can apply into their busy lives.

Intermittent fasting works by eating within a **certain time period** or an **"eating window"** within a day and then fasting (don't eat) for the rest of the day.

For example, let's say you have an "eating window" **Monday - Friday from 11:00 AM – 7:00 PM**.

This means that you can eat (usually 2 meals or more) from **11:00 AM – 7:00 PM**. Once your "eating window" **closes**, you simply fast for the rest of the day.

For example, say you decide to eat an early lunch at **11:30 AM.**

Then, you decide to eat a healthy snack around **2:30 PM**.

You then eat your last meal around **6:00 PM.**

After you finish eating your last meal, your eating window then **closes at 7:00 PM**, which means there is no more eating until the following day.

It is important to state that when you **temporarily fast** (don't eat) for a period of time, you get to experience all kinds of life-changing benefits.

Some of The Benefits of Intermittent Fasting Are:
- You develop **discipline** with your eating habits.

- You will feel more **alert and energetic** while fasting.

- Increases your **life expectancy**.

- Helps you to **lose weight, burn off stubborn belly fat** and reduces your urge for **overeating**.

- Allows you to develop a **flexible** eating schedule around your busy work/life.

- Allows you to eat 2 healthy delicious meals a day (including a snack) giving you more **free time** to focus on other priorities in your life.

Overall, intermittent fasting is a great **tool** that any busy person can use for eating healthy, losing belly fat quickly and staying fit.

#4 Use A Food Journal

Using a food journal is a great way to **keep track** of all the food you eat on a daily basis.

In addition, using a food journal will help you to **eliminate overeating** as well as help you to **lose belly fat** and keep it off.

When using a food journal, all you have to do is simply **write down** what eat you every day.

Make sure to include any **snacks, teas, coffee and drinks** in your food journal.

Writing down what you eat using a food journal is a **great habit** to develop.

By using a food journal, you will come to realize **how healthy** you are eating as well as become more aware of all the **unhealthy foods** you may also be eating.

In addition, you can look back at the end of the day at your food journal and determine whether you ate too much or not.

If you feel like you are simply eating too much or that you want to lose a **few extra pounds**, you can use your food journal as a way to see what foods you may want to eat less of.

You can use a **notebook, your computer** or even an **online App** as a food journal in order to keep track of the food you eat every day.

At the end of the day, you can refer back to your food journal and ask yourself questions like:

- Did I eat a healthy delicious meal today?
- Did I eat enough fruits and vegetables?
- Did I drink enough water?
- Did I eat any unhealthy foods or snacks?
- Didi I feel extremely full after each meal?
- Did I feel energetic or tired as a result of the foods I ate?

Using a food journal is great for helping you to **keep focused** on your diet.

In addition, a food journal helps you to develop good **eating habits**, provides **motivation** for achieving your health and fitness goals and it is an effective way to simply burn belly fat and lose weight.

#5 Use A Food Scale

Use a food scale to weigh your food before you cook it so that you know exactly **how much food** you will be consuming every day both for lunch and dinner.

By using a food scale, you will also be able to **keep track of the number of calories** you eat every day.

In addition, you will be more efficient at **losing weight** because you will not be **overeating** as a result of **keeping track** of how much food you eat every day.

Research shows that **80% of weight loss** is all about your diet as well as **what you eat and how much you eat.**

So, by weighing your food, you will know if you need to **reduce the number of calories** you are eating in order to lose belly fat.

In addition, weighing your food will help you to **maintain** your desired weight 365 days a year.

Conclusion

You have now learned **5 life-changing tips** for losing belly fat and improving your overall health.

In addition, you have learned about the remarkable **Mediterranean Diet** and its amazing health benefits.

The next step is to **immediately** get started with applying what you have learned into your daily life.

Remember, once you begin to use the valuable information provided in this amazing eBook you will **develop remarkable habits** that will greatly improve your health and your overall life.

I wish you great success on your journey to a **healthier** and **happier** you.

Eberto A. Rios
30DayBellyFatloss.com

For more information about

Weight Loss and Health visit…

https://www.30daybellyfatloss.com/

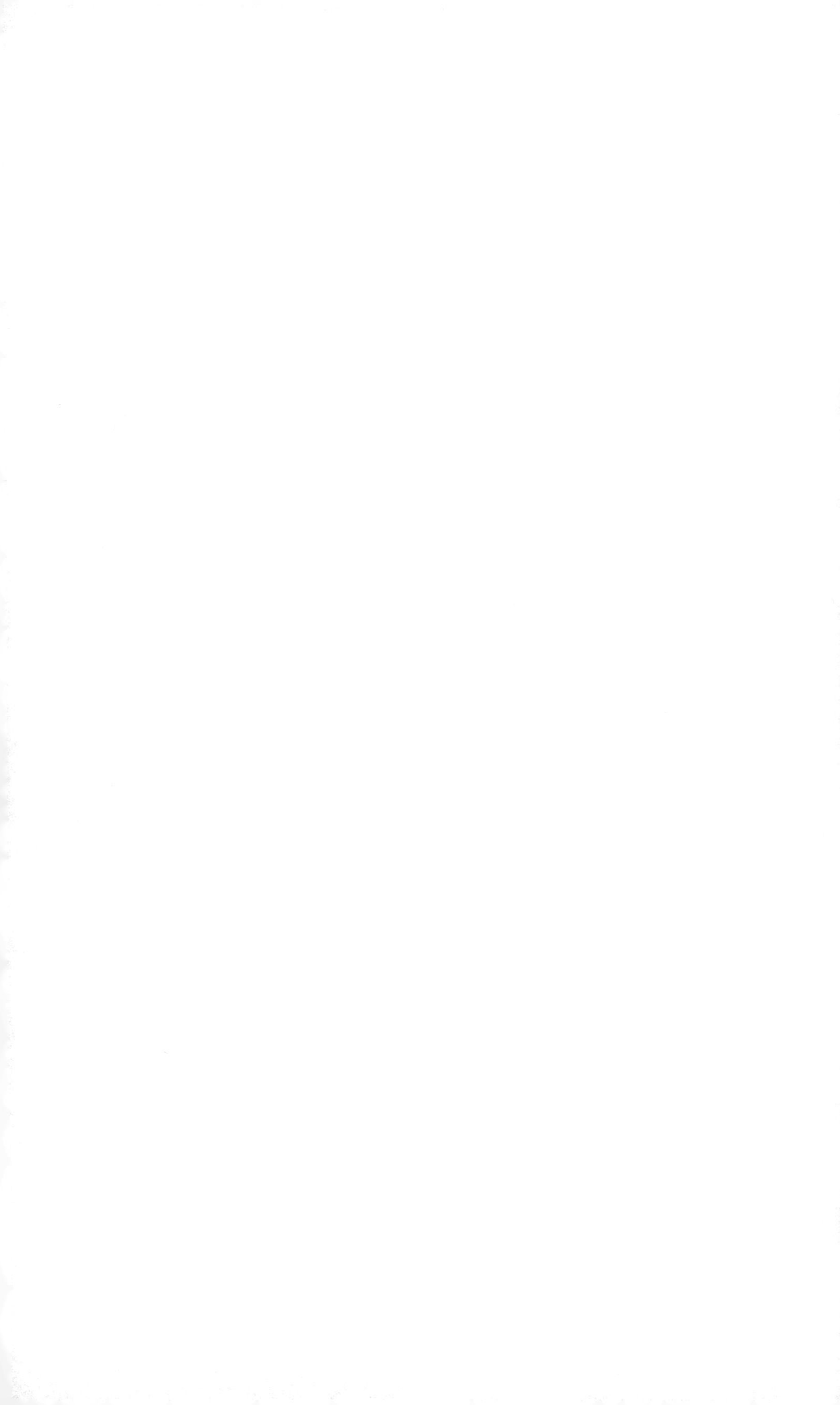

www.ingramcontent.com/pod-product-compliance
Lightning Source LLC
Chambersburg PA
CBHW031228250726
48655CB00005B/1860